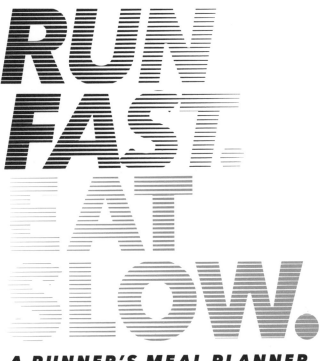

RUN FAST. EAT SLOW.

A RUNNER'S MEAL PLANNER

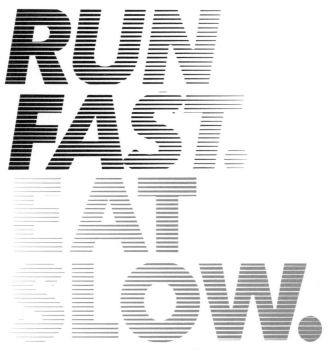

RUN FAST. EAT SLOW.

A RUNNER'S MEAL PLANNER

WITH

52

WEEK-AT-A-GLANCE GRIDS, RECIPES, AND TIPS TO FUEL HAPPY

SHALANE FLANAGAN & ELYSE KOPECKY

CLARKSON POTTER/PUBLISHERS
NEW YORK

All rights reserved.
Published in the United States by Clarkson Potter/
Publishers, an imprint of Random House, a division of
Penguin Random House LLC, New York.
rodalebooks.com

CLARKSON POTTER is a trademark and POTTER with
colophon is a registered trademark of Penguin Random
House LLC.

ISBN 978-1-9848-2652-7

Printed in China

Cover design by Danielle Deschenes
Book design by Rae Ann Spitzenberger

10 9 8 7 6 5 4 3 2 1

First Edition

HI, ATHLETE!

If you've read our best-selling cookbook *Run Fast. Eat Slow.* and its sequel, *Run Fast. Cook Fast. Eat Slow,* you know the Shalane-Elyse mantra. If you haven't read our books, here's what you need to know:

Outside of running more miles, the single greatest thing athletes can do to improve their performances (and their long-term health and happiness) is learn to cook.

Our muscles have been burning (and stomachs growling) since we met on the cross-country team at UNC Chapel Hill nineteen years ago. Shalane went on to become a four-time Olympian. And Elyse went on to culinary-nutrition school, where she learned all about what athletes—particularly women— need to eat to win. (Clue: it's not packaged foods!) Together we conjured *Run Fast. Eat Slow.* after watching so many of our friends and teammates (and ourselves!) suffer from injuries and health issues that could be prevented with proper nutrition.

In this planner, we're extending our mission to inspire athletes of all levels to cook their way to success. Cooking from scratch can be daunting and time consuming, but it need not be. Here, we'll help you get organized and inspire you to plan out your meals so that ingredients get used multiple times and leftovers never go to waste. And our handy meal prep tips will ensure you're always one step ahead of a *hangry* meltdown.

You may see some ideas in here and in our cookbooks that sound unfamiliar—that's because most of the trendy diets pushed at endurance athletes these days focus on calories and macros. That reductive thinking leads to undernourishment, an unhealthy relationship with food, and a general fear of stepping into the kitchen. We want the opposite for you! We hope our journal will keep you inspired in the kitchen and help you discover the joy in cooking (and eating!) that we've found in our own kitchens.

Fuel Happy!

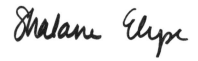

HOW TO USE THIS PLANNER

If you're already planning your training and recording your mileage, you know the benefits of setting goals and sticking to a plan. Similarly, setting aside a half hour every week to plan your meals can save you considerable time and money and prevent headaches in the kitchen.

And this planner is more than a place to record meals. We hope you'll use it as a daily journal and reliable friend. Begin with week 1 whether you start in winter, spring, summer, or fall so you can plan a full year of weekly meals. We've left plenty of room for you to write goals, track runs, jot down recipe notes, record what foods energize you best, or note anything that inspires you.

MEAL PLAN LIKE YOU PLAN YOUR TRAINING

WHY MEAL PLAN?

>> SAVE TIME AND MONEY

By planning your meals for the week, you can do one big grocery run to save time. Fewer trips to the store will also save you money, since you can plan meals back to back that make use of the same ingredients. You'll also know how to repurpose leftovers so that you're not cooking from scratch every single night. If your fridge is well stocked, you'll be less likely to end up at a takeout joint.

A note on organic: we aren't all lucky enough to have access to local farms and farmers' markets—do the best you can and concentrate on finding the freshest produce and, if possible, spend a little extra on organic or free-range eggs, dairy, and meat.

>> LOOK BACK AT THE BEST WEEKS

Did you just have a great week of training or run a PR in a race? Now you'll be able to look back at what you ate that week and see what foods fuel your body best. Recording what you eat will help you see what foods might be causing problems like digestive distress or inflammation.

>> ENJOY COOKING

It's fun to break out a planner, make a cup of your favorite tea, and plot out your meals for the week. Organization is a recipe for success in the kitchen, and success in the kitchen will give you so much pride and enjoyment. Once you smooth out the challenges that keep you from cooking, you will enjoy the process so much more.

>> ELIMINATE FOOD WASTE

Did you know that about 40% of the food produced in the United States is thrown away?! That's an incredible amount of waste of precious resources and has a huge negative impact on our environment. Everyone can do their small part by meal planning to eliminate food waste in their own homes.

>> HEALTH AND HAPPINESS

Delicious homemade food nourishes the mind, body, and soul. We can't think of any undertaking that is a better use of your valuable time (except maybe running!) than cooking real food. It is a crucial element in living an active and happy life. It will give you the energy to go after your crazy dreams.

MEAL PREP LIKE A BOSS

The essential component to meal planning is meal prepping. Meal prepping means cooking dishes or prepping ingredients in advance to stock your fridge. When you come home from a long day and you're feeling "hangry," you'll peek in your fridge and have the components ready to get dinner on the table fast. You'll be a lot less likely to order takeout when dinner is already prepped.

HERE'S HOW IT GOES DOWN IN ELYSE'S KITCHEN . . .

Every Sunday I block out two hours to meal prep for our busy week ahead. As a working mom with two young kids, meal prep is essential to getting dinner on the table fast . . . before the kids get fussy! Meals during the week are simple but nourishing and delicious. Power Bowls (featured in *Run Fast. Cook Fast. Eat Slow.*) are a regular in our household and they usually consist of rice topped with leftover roasted veggies, a fried egg or leftover chicken or steak, sliced avocado, and a homemade sauce or dressing. On Sundays I always roast a big tray of veggies and make a double batch of one of the sauce or dressing recipes in our cookbooks.

Weekly meal prep also includes making a seasonal grain salad or soup with an assortment of seasonal veggies. I pack these hearty grain salads into individual containers for work lunches (like the DIY Grain Salad recipe in *Run Fast. Cook Fast. Eat Slow.*). I typically hard-boil half a dozen eggs for adding on top of lunch salads.

I usually double recipes (especially soups and sauces) so I can stash half in the freezer. I even freeze pesto and homemade hummus. Our family never tires of any of the soup recipes in *Run Fast. Eat Slow*. We'll eat soup for two dinners in a row and, one of the nights, I'll stir in rice or pasta to make it feel like a new meal or add grilled cheese sandwiches or a baguette with butter.

On the weekend, I also bake a wholesome treat like homemade granola or Superhero Muffins for grab-n-go snacks. A Superhero Muffin with a smoothie is our go-to for breakfast on rushed mornings (which is pretty much always during the week!).

The key to making nutrient-dense smoothies every morning is having the ingredients prepped. I freeze bananas and berries, peel carrots, wash greens, and steam beets. Beets are super nutritious and surprisingly versatile for smoothies or salads.

As you'll see in the sample Weekly Meal Plan that follows, I always make good use of leftovers for either lunch or dinner the next day. The mantra in my house is "cook once, eat twice," which saves time, money, and dishes! Cooking an entire meal from scratch night after night can be daunting and overwhelming. You've got my full permission to embrace those leftovers!

Every week I share meal prep tips on Instagram . . . you can follow along for more inspiration @ElyseKopecky.

MAKE TIME TO SAVE TIME

Turn up the music, open a bottle of wine or make a cup of tea, download a favorite podcast, block out your calendar, set your phone to Do Not Disturb mode, get the kids out of the house. Do whatever it takes to dedicate one afternoon per week to meal prep. You'll be a lot less likely to pick up a burrito on the way home from work if you have the quinoa and sauce already made and all you need to do is sauté some chicken and veggies.

5 THINGS TO PREP EVERY WEEK

1 Cook a double batch of whole grains like rice, farro, or quinoa to be used for grain salads, rice bowls, or side dishes.

2 Make a homemade sauce and/or dressing for bowls and salads.

3 Roast a tray (or two!) of mixed seasonal veggies like carrots, cauliflower, potatoes, sweet potatoes, or butternut squash. Roasted veggies are one of the most versatile components to stash in your fridge. Think toppings for pizza night, fillings for Taco Tuesday, toppings for rice bowls, quick side dishes, fillings for omelets and frittatas (see page 68), mix-ins for salads or pasta dishes, and many more possibilities.

4 Make a soup (winter) or a hearty salad (summer). If you're feeding a hungry family, always double your favorite soup recipes. For inspiration, see the recipes after each seasonal opener, which always include seasonal soups and salads.

5 Prep healthy snacks like hummus and veggies, hard-boiled eggs, bags of trail mix, or bake a wholesome treat like Superhero Muffins (recipe page 13), breakfast cookies, or granola. Shalane's go-to snacks, prepped on Sundays, include homemade energy balls (we're obsessed with the Chocolate-Matcha Energy Balls in *Run Fast. Cook Fast. Eat Slow.*) and smoothie ingredients.

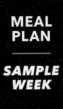

	SUNDAY	MONDAY	TUESDAY
BREAKFAST	>> Homemade pancakes with nut butter >> Sliced banana >> Coffee	>> Pineapple Beet Smoothie **(p. 125)** >> Leftover pancakes >> Coffee	>> Strawberry Beet Oatmeal Bake **(p. 69)** topped with whole-milk yogurt and honey >> Coffee
LUNCH	>> Thai Red Lentil Soup **(p. 183)** >> Tortilla chips >> Fruit	>> Leftover Butternut and Kale Frittata **(p. 181)** >> Leftover soup >> Baguette with butter	>> Leftover Butternut and Kale Frittata **(p. 181)** >> Leftover salad
SNACK	>> Homemade trail mix with nuts, seeds, pretzels, dark chocolate chips >> Green tea	>> Homemade trail mix with nuts, seeds, pretzels, dark chocolate chips >> Green tea	>> Apple or banana with nut butter >> Runner's Recovery Tea
DINNER	>> Butternut and Kale Frittata **(p. 181)** >> Salad with beets, walnuts, feta, homemade dressing	>> Grilled or baked wild salmon >> Hearty seasonal salad (Mighty Cobb; Wild Rice and Mushroom, **pp. 126, 182)**	>> Leftover salmon >> Roasted cauliflower and potatoes >> Sautéed greens
SNACK	>> Whole-milk yogurt with homemade granola	>> Wholesome treat >> Herbal tea	>> Whole-milk yogurt with homemade granola
	DISTANCE _____ TIME _____	DISTANCE _____ TIME _____	DISTANCE _____ TIME _____

WEDNESDAY	THURSDAY	FRIDAY	SATURDAY
>> Whole-milk yogurt with homemade granola or muesli, chopped apple or berries >> Coffee	>> Leftover Strawberry Beet Oatmeal Bake *(p. 69)* topped with whole-milk yogurt >> Coffee	>> Banana Chocolate Superhero Muffin *(p. 13)* >> Hard-boiled egg >> Coffee	>> Omelet with spinach and feta >> Leftover sweet potatoes >> Seasonal fruit >> Coffee
>> Leftover hearty salad topped with hard-boiled egg	>> Leftover soup >> Tortilla chips	>> Fave sandwich >> Leftover soup	>> Fave sandwich or grain salad >> Carrots and hummus
>> Half avocado with sea salt >> Dark chocolate square >> Runner's Recovery Tea	>> Banana Chocolate Superhero Muffin *(p. 13)* >> Chai tea	>> Carrots and hummus >> Fruit >> Green tea	>> Pineapple Beet Smoothie *(p. 125)* >> Pretzels and almonds >> Chai tea
>> Mexican Chicken Soup with Greens *(p. 15)*, toppings >> Simple salad	>> Grass-fed burgers >> Sweet potato fries >> Salad	>> Rice bowl topped with leftover burger, roasted or grilled veggies, guacamole or hummus	>> Sheet-Pan Chicken, Asparagus, and Purple Potatoes *(p. 71)* >> Simple salad
>> Wholesome treat >> Herbal tea	>> Nuts and fruit	>> Homemade apple crumble with yogurt or ice cream	>> Homemade apple crumble with yogurt or ice cream
DISTANCE _____ TIME _____	DISTANCE _____ TIME _____	DISTANCE _____ TIME _____	DISTANCE _____ TIME _____

WINTER

THIS IS THE TIME OF YEAR TO HUNKER DOWN, WEAR
leggings and chunky sweaters, and cook! When the days
get shorter, we become serious homebodies . . . when
we're not charging through rain, sleet, and snow for
exercise. This is the most important time to stock the
larder and fridge so that when you're back from your chilly
adventures and hunger strikes, you've got everything you
need for a soul-warming soup or freshly baked treat
(because the last thing you're going to feel like doing is
venturing back out to go to the grocery store).

WHAT'S COOKING?

Bring on the chili cook-off! We love to make chili, soups,
and stews when the temperatures drop. In the winter
months, it's important to eat more warming foods (less raw
food), which are easier to digest and extremely comforting.
Soups are a great way to pack in immune-boosting
ingredients, since they're loaded with veggies. But don't
completely forget the raw stuff—salad and smoothies,
etc.—as raw fruits and veggies provide the enzymes that
your body needs for optimal digestion. Breakfast should
be a celebration (you got out of that warm bed!): we like
steaming bowls of oatmeal loaded with delicious toppings
like cinnamon, maple syrup, and/or apples sautéed in butter.

FAVE SEASONAL INGREDIENTS

>> Dark Leafy
   Greens
>> Potatoes and Yams

>> Winter Squash
>> Citrus
>> Garlic and Onions

>> Carrots
>> Cauliflower
>> Beets

BANANA *CHOCOLATE*
SUPERHERO MUFFINS

Superhero Muffins have gained celebrity status on social media for good reason. They provide the ideal balance of energizing fats, complex carbs, and protein for breakfast on the go. In Run Fast. Cook Fast. Eat Slow. *we created three new flavors of these muffins, but we couldn't stop there. This antioxidant-rich chocolate flavor just might be our new favorite!* **MAKES 12 MUFFINS**

2 cups almond meal

1½ cups old-fashioned rolled oats

¼ cup unsweetened cocoa powder

1 teaspoon baking soda

½ teaspoon fine sea salt

½ cup chocolate chips

3 large eggs

1½ cups very ripe mashed banana (2 large or 3 medium bananas)

½ cup grated carrot, optional

6 tablespoons unsalted butter, melted

¼ cup honey

1 Position a rack in the center of the oven. Preheat the oven to 350°F. Line a 12-cup standard muffin tin with paper muffin cups.

2 In a large bowl, combine the almond meal, oats, cocoa powder, baking soda, salt, and chocolate chips.

3 In a separate bowl, whisk together the eggs, banana, carrot (if using), melted butter, and honey. Add to the dry ingredients, mixing until combined.

4 Spoon the batter into the muffin cups, filling each to the brim. Bake until the muffins are nicely browned on top and a knife inserted in the center of a muffin comes out clean, 30 to 35 minutes.

5 Store leftover muffins in an airtight container in the fridge or freezer. If you like them warm, reheat on low power in the microwave.

GLUTEN-FREE: Use certified gluten-free oats

VEGGIE *AND* SAUSAGE SKILLET HASH

We're fans of dinners that can be transformed into breakfast the next day, especially when they're hearty and flavor-forward like this skillet hash. Go next level by topping it with an oozy fried egg and sliced avocado. **SERVES 4**

1 tablespoon extra-virgin olive oil

½ yellow onion, diced

¾ pound bulk Italian sausage (without casing)

1 small sweet potato (yam), diced

1 small Yukon Gold potato, diced extra-small (see Note)

½ teaspoon fine sea salt

¼ teaspoon red pepper flakes, optional

1 red bell pepper, seeds removed, diced

2 cups chopped kale

4 eggs, optional

NOTE: *Dice the Yukon Gold potato extra-small to decrease the cook time, since white potatoes take longer to cook than sweet potatoes.*

1 Heat the oil in a large cast-iron or nonstick skillet over medium heat (a 12-inch skillet with a lid, like a Le Creuset Braiser, is ideal). Add the onion and sausage and use a wooden spatula to break them up into bite-size pieces. Cook for 3 minutes, until lightly browned. Keep the fat in the pan (if your sausage is lean you may need to add another tablespoon of oil).

2 Add the sweet potato, Yukon Gold potato, salt, and red pepper flakes (if using) to the skillet. Cover and cook for 15 minutes, stirring every 5 minutes. Add the bell pepper. Cook, uncovered, for 10 to 15 minutes, stirring occasionally, until the potatoes are soft. Add the kale and cook just until wilted.

3 In a separate skillet, fry the eggs according to your preference.

4 Spoon the sausage and veggies into individual bowls and serve topped with a fried egg.

GLUTEN-FREE // DAIRY-FREE // VEG: Sub marinated tempeh

MEXICAN CHICKEN SOUP
WITH GREENS

You can't go wrong with chicken soup, especially when it's topped with avocado, tortilla chips, and melted cheese. We often double this recipe since it makes for easy leftovers for lunch or dinner. **SERVES 5**

2 tablespoons extra-virgin olive oil

2 carrots, peeled and diced

2 celery stalks, diced

1 small yellow onion, diced

1 red bell pepper, diced

1 teaspoon fine sea salt (reduce in half if broth is not low-sodium), plus more as needed

4 garlic cloves, minced

2 tablespoons chili powder

1/4 teaspoon ground cayenne or chipotle pepper, optional

1 box (32 ounces) low-sodium chicken broth

1 pound skinless, boneless chicken thighs

1 can (15 ounces) black beans, rinsed and drained

1 can (15 ounces) diced tomatoes

2 cups chopped greens (kale, spinach, or Swiss chard)

Freshly ground black pepper

TOPPINGS: lime wedges, cilantro, chopped avocado, grated cheddar cheese, crushed tortilla chips

1 Heat the oil in a large pot over medium heat. Add the carrots, celery, onion, bell pepper, and salt, and sauté until softened, about 5 minutes. Add the garlic, chili powder, and cayenne (if using), and sauté for 1 minute.

2 Add the broth, chicken, beans, and tomatoes. Bring to a boil, then turn the heat to low and simmer covered for 30 minutes.

3 Remove the chicken to a cutting board and use two forks to shred it. Return the chicken to the pot along with the greens. Simmer for 5 minutes. Remove from the heat. Taste and add salt and pepper if needed.

4 Ladle into soup bowls and serve with a fun assortment of toppings (see suggestions in the ingredient list).

GLUTEN-FREE // DAIRY-FREE

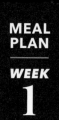

MEAL PLAN

WEEK
1

	SUNDAY	MONDAY	TUESDAY
BREAKFAST			
LUNCH			
SNACK			
DINNER			
SNACK			
	DISTANCE _____ TIME _____	DISTANCE _____ TIME _____	DISTANCE _____ TIME _____

WEDNESDAY	THURSDAY	FRIDAY	SATURDAY
DISTANCE _____ TIME _____	DISTANCE _____ TIME _____	DISTANCE _____ TIME _____	DISTANCE _____ TIME _____

NOTES/
GOALS
WEEK 1

Life and the marathon are a series of ups and downs. Embrace those ups and just muscle through the downs.

—SHALANE

	SUNDAY	MONDAY	TUESDAY
BREAKFAST			
LUNCH			
SNACK			
DINNER			
SNACK			
	DISTANCE _____ TIME _____	DISTANCE _____ TIME _____	DISTANCE _____ TIME _____

WEDNESDAY	THURSDAY	FRIDAY	SATURDAY
DISTANCE _____ TIME _____	DISTANCE _____ TIME _____	DISTANCE _____ TIME _____	DISTANCE _____ TIME _____

NOTES/ GOALS
WEEK 2

My kitchen is always a mess, but at least my family is eating a home-cooked meal every night.
—ELYSE

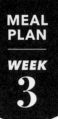

MEAL PLAN

WEEK 3

	SUNDAY	MONDAY	TUESDAY
BREAKFAST			
LUNCH			
SNACK			
DINNER			
SNACK			
	DISTANCE _____ TIME _____	DISTANCE _____ TIME _____	DISTANCE _____ TIME _____

WEDNESDAY	THURSDAY	FRIDAY	SATURDAY
DISTANCE _____ TIME _____	DISTANCE _____ TIME _____	DISTANCE _____ TIME _____	DISTANCE _____ TIME _____

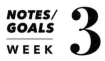

NOTES/ GOALS

WEEK **3**

When in doubt, make Superhero Muffins.

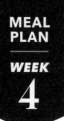

MEAL PLAN

WEEK 4

	SUNDAY	MONDAY	TUESDAY
BREAKFAST			
LUNCH			
SNACK			
DINNER			
SNACK			
	DISTANCE _____ TIME _____	DISTANCE _____ TIME _____	DISTANCE _____ TIME _____

WEDNESDAY	THURSDAY	FRIDAY	SATURDAY
DISTANCE _____ TIME _____	DISTANCE _____ TIME _____	DISTANCE _____ TIME _____	DISTANCE _____ TIME _____

Meal prepping is my lifeline for surviving busy weeknights.

—ELYSE

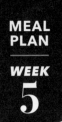

MEAL PLAN

WEEK 5

	SUNDAY	MONDAY	TUESDAY
BREAKFAST			
LUNCH			
SNACK			
DINNER			
SNACK			
	DISTANCE _____ TIME _____	DISTANCE _____ TIME _____	DISTANCE _____ TIME _____

WEDNESDAY	THURSDAY	FRIDAY	SATURDAY
DISTANCE _____ TIME _____	DISTANCE _____ TIME _____	DISTANCE _____ TIME _____	DISTANCE _____ TIME _____

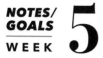

NOTES/ GOALS

WEEK 5

One of the best gifts I've been given to enhance my running career and overall well-being
has been learning to cook.

–SHALANE

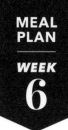

MEAL PLAN

WEEK
6

	SUNDAY	MONDAY	TUESDAY
BREAKFAST			
LUNCH			
SNACK			
DINNER			
SNACK			
	DISTANCE _____ **TIME** _____	**DISTANCE** _____ **TIME** _____	**DISTANCE** _____ **TIME** _____

WEDNESDAY	THURSDAY	FRIDAY	SATURDAY
DISTANCE _____ TIME _____	DISTANCE _____ TIME _____	DISTANCE _____ TIME _____	DISTANCE _____ TIME _____

NOTES/ GOALS
WEEK 6

DATE ___/___/___

Unburden and indulge yourself in our delicious recipes and set audacious goals that will fuel your soul!

—SHALANE

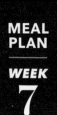

MEAL PLAN

WEEK 7

	SUNDAY	MONDAY	TUESDAY
BREAKFAST			
LUNCH			
SNACK			
DINNER			
SNACK			
	DISTANCE _____ TIME _____	DISTANCE _____ TIME _____	DISTANCE _____ TIME _____

WEDNESDAY	THURSDAY	FRIDAY	SATURDAY
DISTANCE _____ TIME _____	DISTANCE _____ TIME _____	DISTANCE _____ TIME _____	DISTANCE _____ TIME _____

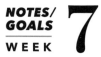

NOTES/ GOALS

WEEK **7**

A setback is just a setup for a comeback.

–SHALANE

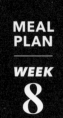

MEAL PLAN

WEEK

8

	SUNDAY	MONDAY	TUESDAY
BREAKFAST			
LUNCH			
SNACK			
DINNER			
SNACK			
	DISTANCE _____ TIME _____	DISTANCE _____ TIME _____	DISTANCE _____ TIME _____

WEDNESDAY	THURSDAY	FRIDAY	SATURDAY

| DISTANCE _____ | DISTANCE _____ | DISTANCE _____ | DISTANCE _____ |
| TIME _____ | TIME _____ | TIME _____ | TIME _____ |

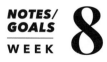

NOTES/
GOALS
WEEK 8

If you're running tense, you're fighting the flow. Relax your jaw and the rest of your body will relax.

—SHALANE

	SUNDAY	MONDAY	TUESDAY
BREAKFAST			
LUNCH			
SNACK			
DINNER			
SNACK			
	DISTANCE _____ TIME _____	DISTANCE _____ TIME _____	DISTANCE _____ TIME _____

WEDNESDAY	THURSDAY	FRIDAY	SATURDAY
DISTANCE _____ TIME _____	DISTANCE _____ TIME _____	DISTANCE _____ TIME _____	DISTANCE _____ TIME _____

Since adding more fat and whole foods into my diet, my racing weight now comes naturally—without counting calories. Hallelujah!!!!

—SHALANE

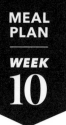

MEAL PLAN

WEEK 10

	SUNDAY	MONDAY	TUESDAY
BREAKFAST			
LUNCH			
SNACK			
DINNER			
SNACK			
	DISTANCE _____ TIME _____	DISTANCE _____ TIME _____	DISTANCE _____ TIME _____

WEDNESDAY	THURSDAY	FRIDAY	SATURDAY
DISTANCE _____ TIME _____	DISTANCE _____ TIME _____	DISTANCE _____ TIME _____	DISTANCE _____ TIME _____

NOTES/ GOALS
WEEK 10

This indulgent diet that I had learned to label in our country as unhealthy actually made me stronger, happier, and healthier than ever before.

—ELYSE

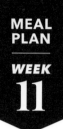

MEAL PLAN

WEEK
11

	SUNDAY	MONDAY	TUESDAY
BREAKFAST			
LUNCH			
SNACK			
DINNER			
SNACK			
	DISTANCE _____ TIME _____	DISTANCE _____ TIME _____	DISTANCE _____ TIME _____

WEDNESDAY	THURSDAY	FRIDAY	SATURDAY
DISTANCE _____ TIME _____	DISTANCE _____ TIME _____	DISTANCE _____ TIME _____	DISTANCE _____ TIME _____

Motherhood is the most rewarding accomplishment of my life. I'm so grateful to have this opportunity to help other women nourish their bodies.

– ELYSE

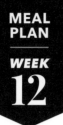

MEAL PLAN

WEEK
12

	SUNDAY	MONDAY	TUESDAY
BREAKFAST			
LUNCH			
SNACK			
DINNER			
SNACK			
	DISTANCE _____ TIME _____	DISTANCE _____ TIME _____	DISTANCE _____ TIME _____

WEDNESDAY	THURSDAY	FRIDAY	SATURDAY
DISTANCE _____ TIME _____	DISTANCE _____ TIME _____	DISTANCE _____ TIME _____	DISTANCE _____ TIME _____

Healthy eating isn't just kale juice, but also a juicy burger.

—ELYSE

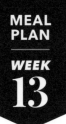

MEAL PLAN

WEEK 13

	SUNDAY	MONDAY	TUESDAY
BREAKFAST			
LUNCH			
SNACK			
DINNER			
SNACK			
	DISTANCE _____ TIME _____	DISTANCE _____ TIME _____	DISTANCE _____ TIME _____

WEDNESDAY	THURSDAY	FRIDAY	SATURDAY
DISTANCE _____ TIME _____	DISTANCE _____ TIME _____	DISTANCE _____ TIME _____	DISTANCE _____ TIME _____

Outside of running more miles, the single greatest thing athletes can do to improve their performance (and their long-term health and happiness) is learn to cook.

–ELYSE

SPRING

IF YOU TEND TO HUNKER DOWN IN THE WINTER, SPRING IS the season to come out of hiding and get amped to increase your mileage. That means as you get back into a running rhythm your kitchen output needs to match your bigger appetite. The more you run, the more nutrition your body will demand. If you find yourself craving late-night sweets and snacks, that's a sign that you aren't fueling right throughout the day. Spring foods should be rejuvenating and refreshing to inspire you to take on a new challenge.

WHAT'S COOKING?

A big breakfast is essential to stay energized all day. In the spring, we're craving omelets filled with the season's first fresh produce. Think asparagus, spinach, and herbs or honey-sweetened strawberry rhubarb sauce over yogurt or oats. For lunch we keep things simple: refreshing salads and thick slices of freshly baked bread with butter. For dinner we're still craving hot meals like pesto pasta (see page 70), rice bowls, salmon, roasted potatoes, and Sheet-Pan Chicken, Asparagus, and Purple Potatoes (page 71).

FAVE SEASONAL INGREDIENTS

>> Asparagus

>> Arugula

>> Strawberries

>> Rhubarb

>> Garlic

>> New Potatoes

>> Fresh Herbs
(tarragon,
parsley, cilantro)

>> Peas

>> Spinach

>> Salad Greens

STRAWBERRY *BEET* OATMEAL BAKE

This supreme solution for make-ahead oatmeal is full of so much goodness. We love that it can be sliced and served like coffee cake, and it's easily reheated for leftovers. Kids will like the burst of color from the beets and berries. Serve topped with plain whole-milk yogurt and an extra drizzle of honey. **SERVES 6**

2 cups old-fashioned rolled oats

¼ cup ground flax seed

1 teaspoon baking powder

1 teaspoon ground cinnamon

¼ teaspoon fine sea salt

1½ cups whole milk or unsweetened nut milk

2 eggs

2 tablespoons unsalted butter, melted, plus more for greasing

2 tablespoons honey or maple syrup

1 teaspoon pure vanilla extract

1 heaping cup chopped fresh strawberries

½ cup grated raw beet (about 1 small beet)

½ cup walnuts, chopped (optional)

1 Preheat the oven to 400°F. Grease an 8 × 8-inch baking dish with butter.

2 In a large bowl, combine the oats, flax seed, baking powder, cinnamon, and salt.

3 In a separate large bowl, whisk together the milk, eggs, melted butter, honey or syrup, and vanilla. Add the wet ingredients to the dry and stir to combine. Stir in the strawberries, beet, and walnuts (if using).

4 Pour into the prepared baking dish and bake in the center of the oven for 40 to 45 minutes, or until set in the middle.

5 Allow to cool and cut into squares. Serve topped with yogurt and a drizzle of honey or maple syrup.

GLUTEN-FREE // DAIRY-FREE: Use nut milk and sub coconut oil

BROCCOLI PESTO LINGUINE

When you have a craving for pasta, we say eat real pasta! Especially if it's our weeknight pesto pasta, which comes together quickly once you get in the habit of stocking your freezer with homemade pesto. We love that this satisfying vegetarian pasta dish can be made in just one pot to save time and dishes. **SERVES 3**

½ box (8 ounces) linguine or spaghetti

1 large or 2 small heads broccoli, cut into florets

¾ cup Presto Pesto (recipe follows) or store-bought

¼ cup chopped kalamata olives (optional)

Freshly ground black pepper, to taste

Grated Parmesan, for serving

PROTEIN BOOST:
This pasta is also delish tossed with sautéed shrimp or leftover grilled chicken.

1 Bring a large pot of salted water to a boil. Cook the pasta according to the package directions until al dente. Reserve ½ cup of the pasta cooking water (don't forget this step!). Drain the pasta and set aside.

2 Add the reserved pasta cooking water back into the pot and bring to a simmer. Add the broccoli, cover, and cook for 4 minutes.

3 Reduce the heat to low. Add the pesto, pasta, olives (if using), and pepper, and stir until just combined and heated through.

4 Top with the grated Parmesan. This dish is best served immediately.

PRESTO PESTO

MAKES 2 CUPS

2 cups tightly packed basil or arugula

6-ounce wedge Parmesan, rind removed, quartered

½ cup toasted walnuts or almonds

1 garlic clove

½ cup extra-virgin olive oil

¼ cup freshly squeezed lemon juice

½ teaspoon fine sea salt

1 In a food processor or high-speed blender, combine the basil or arugula, Parmesan, nuts, and garlic. Pulse until finely ground. Add the oil, lemon juice, and salt. Process until smooth, scraping down the sides as needed until fully blended.

2 Transfer to a wide-mouthed glass jar and store in the refrigerator for up to 5 days.

VEGETARIAN

SHEET-PAN CHICKEN, ASPARAGUS, *AND* PURPLE POTATOES

On busy weeknights, sheet-pan complete meals are your new bestie. When you're maxing out your mileage, chicken and potatoes are a steadfast and easy-to-digest combo to replenish your depleted protein and glycogen stores. **SERVES 4**

2½ pounds (about 6 pieces) bone-in, skin-on chicken thighs

1 teaspoon fine sea salt

Freshly ground black pepper

1½ pounds purple potatoes (or other small variety), chopped into bite-size pieces

2 tablespoons extra-virgin olive oil

1 bunch of asparagus, ends trimmed, cut into thirds (see Note)

3 small shallots, peeled and quartered, ends trimmed

½ teaspoon garlic powder

½ teaspoon smoked paprika

1 Preheat the oven to 425°F and line a rimmed baking sheet with parchment paper.

2 Arrange the chicken thighs on a plate, pat dry with a paper towel, and sprinkle on all sides with ½ teaspoon of the salt and a generous amount of black pepper. Set aside.

3 Place the potatoes on the baking sheet and toss with the olive oil and the remaining ½ teaspoon of salt. Roast in the center of the oven for 15 minutes.

4 Remove from the oven and toss with the asparagus, shallots, garlic powder, and paprika.

5 Spread the vegetables out on the baking sheet and nestle the chicken on top with skin side up.

6 Roast in the center of the oven about 30 minutes, until the chicken is cooked through and has reached an internal temperature of 165°F.

NOTE: *When asparagus is not in season, you can substitute Brussels sprouts, broccoli, or cauliflower.*

GLUTEN-FREE // DAIRY-FREE

MEAL PLAN

WEEK
14

	SUNDAY	MONDAY	TUESDAY
BREAKFAST			
LUNCH			
SNACK			
DINNER			
SNACK			
	DISTANCE _____ TIME _____	DISTANCE _____ TIME _____	DISTANCE _____ TIME _____

WEDNESDAY	THURSDAY	FRIDAY	SATURDAY
DISTANCE _____ TIME _____	DISTANCE _____ TIME _____	DISTANCE _____ TIME _____	DISTANCE _____ TIME _____

NOTES/ GOALS
WEEK 14

Get ready to fuel your best life.

—RUN FAST. EAT SLOW.

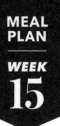

MEAL PLAN

WEEK 15

	SUNDAY	MONDAY	TUESDAY
BREAKFAST			
LUNCH			
SNACK			
DINNER			
SNACK			
	DISTANCE _____ TIME _____	DISTANCE _____ TIME _____	DISTANCE _____ TIME _____

WEDNESDAY	THURSDAY	FRIDAY	SATURDAY
DISTANCE _____ TIME _____	DISTANCE _____ TIME _____	DISTANCE _____ TIME _____	DISTANCE _____ TIME _____

NOTES/ GOALS
WEEK 15

Whether you're a beginner training for your first 5K and trying to shed a few pounds or an elite athlete training for a marathon, you need healthy fats in your life.

−RUN FAST. EAT SLOW.

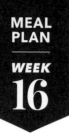

MEAL PLAN

WEEK 16

	SUNDAY	MONDAY	TUESDAY
BREAKFAST			
LUNCH			
SNACK			
DINNER			
SNACK			
	DISTANCE _____ TIME _____	DISTANCE _____ TIME _____	DISTANCE _____ TIME _____

WEDNESDAY	THURSDAY	FRIDAY	SATURDAY
DISTANCE _____ TIME _____	DISTANCE _____ TIME _____	DISTANCE _____ TIME _____	DISTANCE _____ TIME _____

NOTES/ GOALS
WEEK 16

Instead of following rules, we want to teach you to get back in tune with listening to your body's hunger signals.

—RUN FAST. EAT SLOW.

	SUNDAY	MONDAY	TUESDAY
BREAKFAST			
LUNCH			
SNACK			
DINNER			
SNACK			
	DISTANCE _____ TIME _____	DISTANCE _____ TIME _____	DISTANCE _____ TIME _____

WEDNESDAY	THURSDAY	FRIDAY	SATURDAY
DISTANCE _____ TIME _____	DISTANCE _____ TIME _____	DISTANCE _____ TIME _____	DISTANCE _____ TIME _____

NOTES/ GOALS
WEEK 17

MEAL PLAN

WEEK
18

	SUNDAY	MONDAY	TUESDAY
BREAKFAST			
LUNCH			
SNACK			
DINNER			
SNACK			
	DISTANCE _____ TIME _____	DISTANCE _____ TIME _____	DISTANCE _____ TIME _____

WEDNESDAY	THURSDAY	FRIDAY	SATURDAY
DISTANCE _____ TIME _____	DISTANCE _____ TIME _____	DISTANCE _____ TIME _____	DISTANCE _____ TIME _____

A diet rich in whole-food fats (even saturated fat) is essential for a healthy metabolism, balanced hormones, and satiation—all of which prevent weight gain.

–RUN FAST. EAT SLOW.

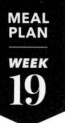

	SUNDAY	MONDAY	TUESDAY
BREAKFAST			
LUNCH			
SNACK			
DINNER			
SNACK			
	DISTANCE _____ TIME _____	DISTANCE _____ TIME _____	DISTANCE _____ TIME _____

WEDNESDAY	THURSDAY	FRIDAY	SATURDAY
DISTANCE _____ TIME _____	DISTANCE _____ TIME _____	DISTANCE _____ TIME _____	DISTANCE _____ TIME _____

Spend more time pursuing your favorite athletic endeavors and less time stressing about what's for breakfast, lunch, and dinner.

—RUN FAST. EAT SLOW.

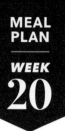

MEAL
PLAN

WEEK
20

	SUNDAY	MONDAY	TUESDAY
BREAKFAST			
LUNCH			
SNACK			
DINNER			
SNACK			
	DISTANCE _____ TIME _____	DISTANCE _____ TIME _____	DISTANCE _____ TIME _____

WEDNESDAY	THURSDAY	FRIDAY	SATURDAY
DISTANCE _____ TIME _____	DISTANCE _____ TIME _____	DISTANCE _____ TIME _____	DISTANCE _____ TIME _____

DATE ___/___/___

If Shalane can whip up rice bowls with roasted veggies, grilled chicken, and homemade sauce after a 20-mile training run, you, too, can dig deep and find the energy to get into the kitchen.

—ELYSE

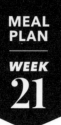

MEAL PLAN

WEEK
21

	SUNDAY	MONDAY	TUESDAY
BREAKFAST			
LUNCH			
SNACK			
DINNER			
SNACK			
	DISTANCE _____ TIME _____	DISTANCE _____ TIME _____	DISTANCE _____ TIME _____

WEDNESDAY	THURSDAY	FRIDAY	SATURDAY
DISTANCE _____ TIME _____	DISTANCE _____ TIME _____	DISTANCE _____ TIME _____	DISTANCE _____ TIME _____

Eating healthy is expensive. But you're worth it. Think of it as an investment in your future self.

–RUN FAST. EAT SLOW.

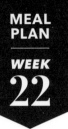

MEAL PLAN

WEEK
22

	SUNDAY	MONDAY	TUESDAY
BREAKFAST			
LUNCH			
SNACK			
DINNER			
SNACK			
	DISTANCE _____ TIME _____	DISTANCE _____ TIME _____	DISTANCE _____ TIME _____

WEDNESDAY	THURSDAY	FRIDAY	SATURDAY
DISTANCE _____ TIME _____	DISTANCE _____ TIME _____	DISTANCE _____ TIME _____	DISTANCE _____ TIME _____

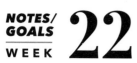

NOTES/ GOALS

WEEK 22

You live a life on the go, and nutritious food can go with you. That food need not be time consuming, bland, or boring.

–RUN FAST. EAT SLOW.

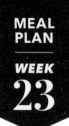

MEAL PLAN

WEEK
23

	SUNDAY	MONDAY	TUESDAY
BREAKFAST			
LUNCH			
SNACK			
DINNER			
SNACK			
	DISTANCE _____ TIME _____	DISTANCE _____ TIME _____	DISTANCE _____ TIME _____

WEEK OF _____ **TO** _____

WEDNESDAY	THURSDAY	FRIDAY	SATURDAY
DISTANCE _____ TIME _____	DISTANCE _____ TIME _____	DISTANCE _____ TIME _____	DISTANCE _____ TIME _____

Nourishing fats are essential for brain function. Studies show that fat helps prevent depression, balances our emotions, and improves concentration.

–RUN FAST. EAT SLOW.

	SUNDAY	MONDAY	TUESDAY
BREAKFAST			
LUNCH			
SNACK			
DINNER			
SNACK			
	DISTANCE _____ TIME _____	DISTANCE _____ TIME _____	DISTANCE _____ TIME _____

WEEK OF _____ TO _____

WEDNESDAY	THURSDAY	FRIDAY	SATURDAY
DISTANCE _____ TIME _____	DISTANCE _____ TIME _____	DISTANCE _____ TIME _____	DISTANCE _____ TIME _____

Meal plan like you plan your training.

—ELYSE

	SUNDAY	MONDAY	TUESDAY
BREAKFAST			
LUNCH			
SNACK			
DINNER			
SNACK			
	DISTANCE _____ TIME _____	DISTANCE _____ TIME _____	DISTANCE _____ TIME _____

WEDNESDAY	THURSDAY	FRIDAY	SATURDAY
DISTANCE _____ TIME _____	DISTANCE _____ TIME _____	DISTANCE _____ TIME _____	DISTANCE _____ TIME _____

DATE ___/___/___

The recipes in Run Fast. Eat Slow. *powered me to achieve my ultimate dream of winning a major marathon. I truly believe cooking wholesome meals will help you win too!*

—SHALANE

	SUNDAY	MONDAY	TUESDAY
BREAKFAST			
LUNCH			
SNACK			
DINNER			
SNACK			
	DISTANCE _____ TIME _____	DISTANCE _____ TIME _____	DISTANCE _____ TIME _____

WEDNESDAY	THURSDAY	FRIDAY	SATURDAY
DISTANCE _____ TIME _____	DISTANCE _____ TIME _____	DISTANCE _____ TIME _____	DISTANCE _____ TIME _____

Focusing on fueling for health and performance is an integral part of my training regimen.

—SHALANE

SUMMER

IN THE SUMMER WE LIKE TO KEEP MEAL PREP AND cooking super simple so that we can spend more time enjoying the sunshine and weekend adventures. Luckily, summer produce is so full of flavor that less is more. You don't even need to turn on your stove or oven to pull off a delicious and nutritious dinner. The key is to stock a high-quality olive oil or pesto to drizzle on everything from tomatoes to refreshing salads to grilled veggies.

WHAT'S COOKING?

We rely on our grills multiple times per week to pull off quick dinners. Examples: grass-fed burgers topped with hummus; fish tacos with mango salsa or guacamole; steak salads; grilled chicken thighs with corn on the cob and summer squash. You can skip marinating your meat when you have our herby Chimichurri (page 127) on hand. The one thing we do use our oven for is sweet potato fries since they pair perfectly with any of the above. For break-fast we rely on yogurt bowls with homemade granola and berries or overnight oats with homemade cashew milk.

A daily fruit and veggie smoothie (see, for example, our Pineapple Beet Smoothie on page 125) is a must-have for hydration and recovery after a sweaty run.

FAVE SEASONAL INGREDIENTS

>> Berries

>> Stone Fruit

>> Tomatoes

>> Bell Peppers

>> Arugula and Salad Greens

>> Fresh Herbs (basil, parsley, mint, cilantro)

>> Zucchini

>> Beets

>> Avocados

>> Green Beans

ANTI-INFLAMMATORY
PINEAPPLE BEET SMOOTHIE

Whipping up a fruit and veggie smoothie is a daily occurrence in our homes for a nourishing start to the day. If you've read Run Fast. Eat Slow., *you know beets are one of our favorite smoothie ingredients. This smoothie just might beet out our famous Can't Beet Me Smoothie for its refreshing tropical flavor.* **SERVES 2**

1 small or ½ large cooked beet, peeled

1 cup frozen pineapple

1 frozen banana

1-inch nob of fresh turmeric, peeled

1-inch nob of fresh ginger, peeled

1 cup coconut water or unsweetened nut milk

1 cup filtered water

2 tablespoons almond butter

2 tablespoons collagen protein (optional)

In a high-speed blender, place the beet, pineapple, banana, turmeric, ginger, coconut water or nut milk, filtered water, almond butter, and collagen protein (if using). Blend on high speed for several minutes until smooth.

GLUTEN-FREE // DAIRY-FREE

MIGHTY **COBB SALAD**

This meal-size power salad is loaded with protein and a quadruple boost of omega-3 fats from the salmon, egg, avocado, and nuts or seeds. It's a simple recovery meal that will keep you satisfied for lunch or dinner. **SERVES 4**

BALSAMIC DRESSING

⅓ cup extra-virgin olive oil

¼ cup balsamic vinegar

1 tablespoon Dijon mustard

Freshly ground black pepper

2 hearts of romaine, chopped

½ head of radicchio, chopped

4 ounces smoked wild salmon (or other protein)

2 hard-boiled eggs, peeled and diced

1 cup halved cherry tomatoes

1 cup chopped green beans (see Note)

1 cup canned chickpeas, rinsed and drained

1 avocado, chopped

½ cup crumbled feta or blue cheese

½ cup chopped walnuts or sunflower seeds

1 In a glass jar with a lid, combine the oil, vinegar, mustard, and pepper. Shake vigorously until emulsified.

2 Combine the lettuces and arrange on a platter. Arrange the toppings in rows on top of the lettuce. Serve with the dressing on the side for drizzling on top.

NOTE: *If you prefer your green beans cooked, simply blanch them in a small pot of boiling water for 2 minutes, transfer to a bowl of ice water to cool, and drain.*

GLUTEN-FREE

CHIMICHURRI

There's no need to marinate your meat when you're serving it slathered with this simple herby sauce. Serve on top of grilled chicken, steak, kebabs, or flaky whitefish. It's got immune-boosting and inflammation-fighting powers, plus a fresh flavor that will keep you coming back for more. **MAKES ¾ CUP**

2 cups fresh herbs (equal combo of parsley, basil, cilantro)

2 tablespoons red wine vinegar

2 garlic cloves

½ teaspoon fine sea salt

Generous pinch of red pepper flakes

½ cup extra-virgin olive oil

In a food processor, combine the herbs, vinegar, garlic, salt, and red pepper. Pulse until the herbs are chopped. Add the olive oil and process until well blended.

GLUTEN-FREE // DAIRY-FREE

	SUNDAY	MONDAY	TUESDAY
BREAKFAST			
LUNCH			
SNACK			
DINNER			
SNACK			
	DISTANCE _____ TIME _____	DISTANCE _____ TIME _____	DISTANCE _____ TIME _____

WEDNESDAY	THURSDAY	FRIDAY	SATURDAY
DISTANCE _____ TIME _____	DISTANCE _____ TIME _____	DISTANCE _____ TIME _____	DISTANCE _____ TIME _____

Celebrate real food for the wealth of benefits it provides for both your body and mind.

–RUN FAST. EAT SLOW.

MEAL PLAN

WEEK
28

	SUNDAY	MONDAY	TUESDAY
BREAKFAST			
LUNCH			
SNACK			
DINNER			
SNACK			
	DISTANCE _____ TIME _____	DISTANCE _____ TIME _____	DISTANCE _____ TIME _____

WEDNESDAY	THURSDAY	FRIDAY	SATURDAY
DISTANCE _____ TIME _____	DISTANCE _____ TIME _____	DISTANCE _____ TIME _____	DISTANCE _____ TIME _____

Maybe you need more butter in your life.

—ELYSE

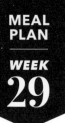

MEAL PLAN

WEEK 29

	SUNDAY	MONDAY	TUESDAY
BREAKFAST			
LUNCH			
SNACK			
DINNER			
SNACK			
	DISTANCE _____ TIME _____	DISTANCE _____ TIME _____	DISTANCE _____ TIME _____

WEDNESDAY	THURSDAY	FRIDAY	SATURDAY
DISTANCE _____ TIME _____	DISTANCE _____ TIME _____	DISTANCE _____ TIME _____	DISTANCE _____ TIME _____

Try to avoid coffee after lunch. It can cause sleep disturbances, and sleep is just as important as nutrition for recovery. Green tea (or a square of dark chocolate!) is a great option if you need a light p.m. caffeine boost.

—RUN FAST. EAT SLOW.

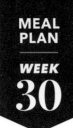

MEAL PLAN

WEEK
30

	SUNDAY	MONDAY	TUESDAY
BREAKFAST			
LUNCH			
SNACK			
DINNER			
SNACK			
	DISTANCE _____ TIME _____	DISTANCE _____ TIME _____	DISTANCE _____ TIME _____

WEDNESDAY	THURSDAY	FRIDAY	SATURDAY
DISTANCE _____ TIME _____	DISTANCE _____ TIME _____	DISTANCE _____ TIME _____	DISTANCE _____ TIME _____

Relax with a cup of herbal tea and a light snack before bed. Our go-to is whole-milk yogurt topped with mineral-rich homemade granola.

—RUN FAST. EAT SLOW.

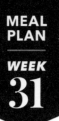

MEAL PLAN

WEEK
31

	SUNDAY	MONDAY	TUESDAY
BREAKFAST			
LUNCH			
SNACK			
DINNER			
SNACK			
	DISTANCE _____ TIME _____	DISTANCE _____ TIME _____	DISTANCE _____ TIME _____

WEDNESDAY	THURSDAY	FRIDAY	SATURDAY
DISTANCE _____ TIME _____	DISTANCE _____ TIME _____	DISTANCE _____ TIME _____	DISTANCE _____ TIME _____

Cook once, eat twice. Leftovers are always celebrated in my home.

—ELYSE

	SUNDAY	MONDAY	TUESDAY
BREAKFAST			
LUNCH			
SNACK			
DINNER			
SNACK			
	DISTANCE _____ TIME _____	DISTANCE _____ TIME _____	DISTANCE _____ TIME _____

WEDNESDAY	THURSDAY	FRIDAY	SATURDAY
DISTANCE _____ TIME _____	DISTANCE _____ TIME _____	DISTANCE _____ TIME _____	DISTANCE _____ TIME _____

NOTES/
GOALS
WEEK 32

In an ordinary training day, I remind myself that I am preparing for the extraordinary.

—SHALANE

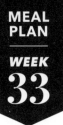

MEAL PLAN

WEEK **33**

	SUNDAY	MONDAY	TUESDAY
BREAKFAST			
LUNCH			
SNACK			
DINNER			
SNACK			
	DISTANCE _____ TIME _____	DISTANCE _____ TIME _____	DISTANCE _____ TIME _____

WEDNESDAY	THURSDAY	FRIDAY	SATURDAY
DISTANCE _____ TIME _____	DISTANCE _____ TIME _____	DISTANCE _____ TIME _____	DISTANCE _____ TIME _____

NOTES/GOALS
WEEK
33

One of my favorite quotes that I always tell myself is "You don't train to feel your best, you train to be at your best when you feel your worst."

—SHALANE

	SUNDAY	MONDAY	TUESDAY
BREAKFAST			
LUNCH			
SNACK			
DINNER			
SNACK			
	DISTANCE _____ TIME _____	DISTANCE _____ TIME _____	DISTANCE _____ TIME _____

WEDNESDAY	THURSDAY	FRIDAY	SATURDAY
DISTANCE _____ TIME _____	DISTANCE _____ TIME _____	DISTANCE _____ TIME _____	DISTANCE _____ TIME _____

NOTES/ GOALS
WEEK 34

In the midst of hard workouts I like to practice pushing through the discomfort and pain I will inevitably feel on race day. I use mantras to help myself focus and live in the moment.

−SHALANE

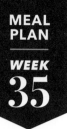

MEAL
PLAN

WEEK
35

	SUNDAY	MONDAY	TUESDAY
BREAKFAST			
LUNCH			
SNACK			
DINNER			
SNACK			
	DISTANCE _____ TIME _____	DISTANCE _____ TIME _____	DISTANCE _____ TIME _____

WEDNESDAY	THURSDAY	FRIDAY	SATURDAY
DISTANCE _____ TIME _____	DISTANCE _____ TIME _____	DISTANCE _____ TIME _____	DISTANCE _____ TIME _____

My race-day breakfast consists of a large bowl of oatmeal with almond milk, honey, walnuts or almonds, bananas, and raspberries or blueberries.

–SHALANE

	SUNDAY	MONDAY	TUESDAY
BREAKFAST			
LUNCH			
SNACK			
DINNER			
SNACK			
	DISTANCE _____ TIME _____	DISTANCE _____ TIME _____	DISTANCE _____ TIME _____

WEDNESDAY	THURSDAY	FRIDAY	SATURDAY
DISTANCE _____ TIME _____	DISTANCE _____ TIME _____	DISTANCE _____ TIME _____	DISTANCE _____ TIME _____

Proper hydration and fuel every day are vital to racing success. Not just eating right in the week leading up to race day.

–SHALANE

	SUNDAY	MONDAY	TUESDAY
BREAKFAST			
LUNCH			
SNACK			
DINNER			
SNACK			
	DISTANCE _____ TIME _____	DISTANCE _____ TIME _____	DISTANCE _____ TIME _____

WEDNESDAY	THURSDAY	FRIDAY	SATURDAY
DISTANCE _____ TIME _____	DISTANCE _____ TIME _____	DISTANCE _____ TIME _____	DISTANCE _____ TIME _____

NOTES/GOALS
WEEK 37

During peak training, cooking wholesome meals helps me recover, makes me happy, and enhances my training.

—SHALANE

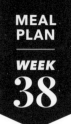

MEAL PLAN

WEEK 38

	SUNDAY	MONDAY	TUESDAY
BREAKFAST			
LUNCH			
SNACK			
DINNER			
SNACK			
	DISTANCE _____ TIME _____	DISTANCE _____ TIME _____	DISTANCE _____ TIME _____

WEDNESDAY	THURSDAY	FRIDAY	SATURDAY
DISTANCE _____ TIME _____	DISTANCE _____ TIME _____	DISTANCE _____ TIME _____	DISTANCE _____ TIME _____

I crave nourishing and salty broths to replenish after a serious sweat session. I like to make a big pot of soup once a week.

−SHALANE

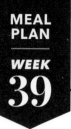

MEAL PLAN

WEEK 39

	SUNDAY	MONDAY	TUESDAY
BREAKFAST			
LUNCH			
SNACK			
DINNER			
SNACK			
	DISTANCE _____ TIME _____	DISTANCE _____ TIME _____	DISTANCE _____ TIME _____

WEDNESDAY	THURSDAY	FRIDAY	SATURDAY
DISTANCE _____	DISTANCE _____	DISTANCE _____	DISTANCE _____
TIME _____	TIME _____	TIME _____	TIME _____

Set goals and share them! I set three goals for every race (in case something goes wrong!): Goals A, B, and C.

—SHALANE

FALL

FALL IS OUR ABSOLUTE FAVORITE TIME OF THE YEAR TO cook! The farmers' market is still going strong, the end of summer produce is full of flavor, the seasonal ingredients are inspiring, and the changing weather gives us an excuse to spend more time in our kitchens.

WHAT'S COOKING?

A mainstay for lunch is hearty grain salads, and for dinner we're devouring rice bowls loaded with roasted fall veggies and a homemade sauce. We don't bake much during the summer, so as soon as the weather cools we enjoy spending more time in the kitchen baking up a storm of homemade goodies. Think granola, muffins, cookies, and apple crisps! We love to make frittatas or egg scrambles with leftover roasted veggies for breakfast, and we're still enjoying our daily smoothie fix.

FAVE SEASONAL INGREDIENTS

- Mushrooms
- Apples and Pears
- End-of-Summer Berries
- Figs
- Butternut Squash
- Cauliflower and Broccoli
- Pumpkin
- Fennel
- Green Beans
- Brussels Sprouts

BUTTERNUT *AND* KALE FRITTATA

The next time you roast a couple of trays of squash or other hearty
veggies like potatoes, set aside 2 cups for a frittata. Frittatas are a
lifeline for busy athletes since they're protein packed and a slice can easily
be reheated to replenish immediately after a hard workout. **SERVES 5**

12 large eggs

½ cup crumbled feta

¼ cup plain whole-milk yogurt

1 teaspoon dried oregano

¼ teaspoon fine sea salt

2 tablespoons extra-virgin olive oil

½ yellow onion, chopped

3 cups chopped kale

2 cups chopped roasted butternut squash (or other roasted veggies)

1 Preheat the oven to 375°F. In a large bowl, whisk together the eggs, feta, yogurt, oregano, and salt. Set aside.

2 Heat the oil in a 12-inch oven-safe skillet over medium-high heat. Add the onion and sauté for 5 minutes. Add the kale and cook just until wilted. Remove the skillet from the heat.

3 Add the squash to the skillet, pour the egg mixture over the top, and lightly stir to evenly spread out the veggies.

4 Bake in the center of the oven for 25 to 30 minutes, or until the eggs have set and the top is golden. Slice and serve.

GLUTEN-FREE

WILD RICE *AND* MUSHROOM SALAD

By planning ahead and cooking a batch of grains on the weekend, you can pull off this satisfying salad for lunch or dinner midweek. Come fall, we crave the earthy flavor of mushrooms. They're high in vitamin D to help us embrace the forthcoming shorter days. **SERVES 5**

2 tablespoons extra-virgin olive oil or butter

4 cups quartered cremini mushrooms (or other variety)

¼ teaspoon fine sea salt

2 cups leftover cooked wild rice, brown rice, or farro, at room temperature

1 apple or pear, cored and chopped

½ cup crumbled feta

6 cups (5 ounces) arugula

⅓ cup chopped toasted walnuts or pecans

DRESSING

⅓ cup extra-virgin olive oil

¼ cup lemon juice or apple cider vinegar

1 tablespoon minced shallot

1 tablespoon honey

1 teaspoon Dijon mustard

¼ teaspoon fine sea salt

1 Heat the oil or butter in a large saucepan or skillet over medium heat. Add the mushrooms and salt. Sauté for 5 minutes, stirring occasionally. Turn the heat to low and cook for 5 to 8 minutes more, stirring occasionally, until tender.

2 Place the dressing ingredients in a glass jar with a lid and shake well to combine.

3 In a medium bowl combine the mushrooms, rice, apple or pear, and feta. Toss with half of the dressing.

4 Arrange the arugula on a large serving platter. Top with the mushroom-rice combo. Top with the nuts. Serve with the remaining dressing on the side for drizzling.

GLUTEN-FREE

THAI RED LENTIL SOUP
WITH COCONUT MILK

This richly satisfying soup promises to warm your soul after a long run in the elements. Feeling fancy? Top each bowl of goodness with toasted pumpkin seeds and roasted cauliflower. Got leftovers? To mix things up, add cooked rice or chicken to the soup the second night. **SERVES 5**

1 tablespoon virgin coconut oil

2 carrots, peeled and chopped

2 celery stalks, chopped

1 yellow onion, chopped

1 teaspoon fine sea salt

2 tablespoons Thai red chili paste

¼ teaspoon ground cayenne, optional (if you like extra heat)

1 box (32 ounces) low-sodium vegetable broth

1½ cups red lentils

1 can (15 ounces) coconut milk (preferably full-fat)

2 to 3 tablespoons freshly squeezed lime juice

Freshly ground black pepper

Toasted pumpkin seeds (optional)

1 Heat the oil in a large pot over medium-high heat. Add the carrots, celery, onion, and salt. Cook, stirring occasionally, until softened but not brown, about 5 minutes. Add the chili paste and cayenne (if using) and stir briefly for 30 seconds, just to coat the veggies.

2 Add the broth, lentils, and coconut milk. Bring to a boil, then reduce the heat and simmer covered, stirring occasionally, until the lentils fall apart, about 30 minutes.

3 Remove the pot from the heat. If you have an immersion (stick) blender, use it to blend the soup right in the pot until smooth. Alternatively, allow the soup to cool slightly, and then transfer it to a blender and process on low until smooth. Please note: Adding hot items to a blender causes the pressure to expand and can blow off the lid, so hold the lid firmly in place and do blend on low.

4 Add the lime juice to taste. Serve topped with black pepper and pumpkin seeds (if using).

VEGAN // GLUTEN-FREE // DAIRY-FREE

MEAL PLAN

WEEK
40

	SUNDAY	MONDAY	TUESDAY
BREAKFAST			
LUNCH			
SNACK			
DINNER			
SNACK			
	DISTANCE _____ TIME _____	DISTANCE _____ TIME _____	DISTANCE _____ TIME _____

WEDNESDAY	THURSDAY	FRIDAY	SATURDAY
DISTANCE _____ TIME _____	DISTANCE _____ TIME _____	DISTANCE _____ TIME _____	DISTANCE _____ TIME _____

NOTES/
GOALS
WEEK
40

The staple workout in my marathon training is the long run. I run anywhere from 20 to 28 miles every 7 to 10 days during my peak season. For those racing shorter distances, like a 5K, their long run might be 8 to 10 miles.

–SHALANE

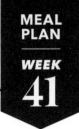

	SUNDAY	MONDAY	TUESDAY
BREAKFAST			
LUNCH			
SNACK			
DINNER			
SNACK			
	DISTANCE _____ TIME _____	DISTANCE _____ TIME _____	DISTANCE _____ TIME _____

WEDNESDAY	THURSDAY	FRIDAY	SATURDAY
DISTANCE _____ TIME _____	DISTANCE _____ TIME _____	DISTANCE _____ TIME _____	DISTANCE _____ TIME _____

Embrace creative leftovers.

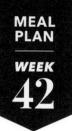

	SUNDAY	MONDAY	TUESDAY
BREAKFAST			
LUNCH			
SNACK			
DINNER			
SNACK			
	DISTANCE _____ TIME _____	DISTANCE _____ TIME _____	DISTANCE _____ TIME _____

WEDNESDAY	THURSDAY	FRIDAY	SATURDAY
DISTANCE _____ TIME _____	DISTANCE _____ TIME _____	DISTANCE _____ TIME _____	DISTANCE _____ TIME _____

While we love cooking, we too don't want to spend all day in the kitchen.

—RUN FAST. EAT SLOW.

	SUNDAY	MONDAY	TUESDAY
BREAKFAST			
LUNCH			
SNACK			
DINNER			
SNACK			
	DISTANCE _____ TIME _____	DISTANCE _____ TIME _____	DISTANCE _____ TIME _____

WEDNESDAY	THURSDAY	FRIDAY	SATURDAY
DISTANCE _____ TIME _____	DISTANCE _____ TIME _____	DISTANCE _____ TIME _____	DISTANCE _____ TIME _____

My training is always enhanced when I share it.

−SHALANE

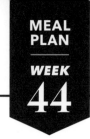

	SUNDAY	MONDAY	TUESDAY
BREAKFAST			
LUNCH			
SNACK			
DINNER			
SNACK			
	DISTANCE _____ TIME _____	DISTANCE _____ TIME _____	DISTANCE _____ TIME _____

WEDNESDAY	THURSDAY	FRIDAY	SATURDAY
DISTANCE _____ TIME _____	DISTANCE _____ TIME _____	DISTANCE _____ TIME _____	DISTANCE _____ TIME _____

NOTES/
GOALS
WEEK 44

A running partner is one of the greatest gifts.

—SHALANE

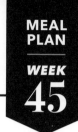

MEAL
PLAN

WEEK
45

	SUNDAY	MONDAY	TUESDAY
BREAKFAST			
LUNCH			
SNACK			
DINNER			
SNACK			
	DISTANCE _____ TIME _____	DISTANCE _____ TIME _____	DISTANCE _____ TIME _____

WEDNESDAY	THURSDAY	FRIDAY	SATURDAY
DISTANCE _____ TIME _____	DISTANCE _____ TIME _____	DISTANCE _____ TIME _____	DISTANCE _____ TIME _____

DATE ___ / ___ / ___

Celebrate real food for the wealth of benefits it provides for both your body and mind.

—ELYSE

MEAL PLAN

WEEK
46

	SUNDAY	MONDAY	TUESDAY
BREAKFAST			
LUNCH			
SNACK			
DINNER			
SNACK			
	DISTANCE _____ TIME _____	DISTANCE _____ TIME _____	DISTANCE _____ TIME _____

WEDNESDAY	THURSDAY	FRIDAY	SATURDAY
DISTANCE _____ TIME _____	DISTANCE _____ TIME _____	DISTANCE _____ TIME _____	DISTANCE _____ TIME _____

Who is your biggest fan? I say be your own biggest fan. Self-belief is powerful.

—SHALANE

MEAL PLAN

WEEK
47

	SUNDAY	MONDAY	TUESDAY
BREAKFAST			
LUNCH			
SNACK			
DINNER			
SNACK			
	DISTANCE _____ TIME _____	DISTANCE _____ TIME _____	DISTANCE _____ TIME _____

WEEK OF _____ TO _____

WEDNESDAY	THURSDAY	FRIDAY	SATURDAY
DISTANCE _____ TIME _____	DISTANCE _____ TIME _____	DISTANCE _____ TIME _____	DISTANCE _____ TIME _____

Overprepare, then go with the flow.

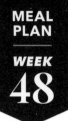

MEAL PLAN

WEEK 48

	SUNDAY	MONDAY	TUESDAY
BREAKFAST			
LUNCH			
SNACK			
DINNER			
SNACK			
	DISTANCE _____ TIME _____	DISTANCE _____ TIME _____	DISTANCE _____ TIME _____

WEDNESDAY	THURSDAY	FRIDAY	SATURDAY
DISTANCE _____ TIME _____	DISTANCE _____ TIME _____	DISTANCE _____ TIME _____	DISTANCE _____ TIME _____

Don't let fear decide your future.

—SHALANE

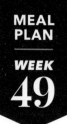

MEAL PLAN

WEEK
49

	SUNDAY	MONDAY	TUESDAY
BREAKFAST			
LUNCH			
SNACK			
DINNER			
SNACK			
	DISTANCE _____ TIME _____	DISTANCE _____ TIME _____	DISTANCE _____ TIME _____

WEDNESDAY	THURSDAY	FRIDAY	SATURDAY
DISTANCE _____ TIME _____	DISTANCE _____ TIME _____	DISTANCE _____ TIME _____	DISTANCE _____ TIME _____

All runners are tough. Everyone has a little fire in them that, even in tough times, can't be turned off.

–SHALANE

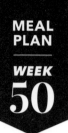

MEAL
PLAN

WEEK
50

	SUNDAY	MONDAY	TUESDAY
BREAKFAST			
LUNCH			
SNACK			
DINNER			
SNACK			
	DISTANCE _____ TIME _____	DISTANCE _____ TIME _____	DISTANCE _____ TIME _____

WEDNESDAY	THURSDAY	FRIDAY	SATURDAY
DISTANCE _____ TIME _____	DISTANCE _____ TIME _____	DISTANCE _____ TIME _____	DISTANCE _____ TIME _____

NOTES/ GOALS
WEEK **50**

DATE ___ / ___ / ___

All macronutrients are not created equal. Judging the health of a food based on how many grams of protein or fat it has is dangerous because these numbers don't reveal the nutrient quality of the food. It's akin to buying a pair of running shoes based solely on their weight without looking at the quality of the technology or considering how the shoe feels on your foot.

—ELYSE

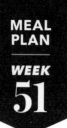

MEAL PLAN

WEEK
51

	SUNDAY	MONDAY	TUESDAY
BREAKFAST			
LUNCH			
SNACK			
DINNER			
SNACK			
	DISTANCE _____ TIME _____	DISTANCE _____ TIME _____	DISTANCE _____ TIME _____

WEDNESDAY	THURSDAY	FRIDAY	SATURDAY
DISTANCE _____	DISTANCE _____	DISTANCE _____	DISTANCE _____
TIME _____	TIME _____	TIME _____	TIME _____

Write down your goals. Share them with friends or family. Be brave enough to go for what you want. Live life with no regrets.

–SHALANE

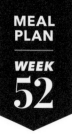

MEAL PLAN

WEEK
52

	SUNDAY	MONDAY	TUESDAY
BREAKFAST			
LUNCH			
SNACK			
DINNER			
SNACK			
	DISTANCE _____ TIME _____	DISTANCE _____ TIME _____	DISTANCE _____ TIME _____

WEDNESDAY	THURSDAY	FRIDAY	SATURDAY
DISTANCE _____ TIME _____	DISTANCE _____ TIME _____	DISTANCE _____ TIME _____	DISTANCE _____ TIME _____

A simple mantra I repeat to myself when I'm struggling on a long run is "Nothing worthwhile ever comes easy."

–SHALANE